FAT LOSS AFTER 40

FAT LOSS AFTER 40+

A SIMPLE SYSTEM TO REDUCE INFLAMMATION, RESET YOUR BODY, AND RESTORE HEALTH

ERIC GUTTMANN

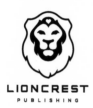

LIONCREST
PUBLISHING

FAT LOSS AFTER 40

A Simple System to Reduce Inflammation,
Reset Your Body, and Restore Health

FIRST EDITION

ISBN   978-1-5445-3390-2 *Hardcover*
        978-1-5445-3392-6 *Paperback*
        978-1-5445-3391-9 *Ebook*

To everyone over forty who wants to lose weight.

This book is for you.

CONTENTS

INTRODUCTION

D.R. had a successful business, and during the editing of one of his promotional videos, he saw what he called a "disgusting fat guy in the video."

Turns out it was *him!*

He was in his late forties with an extra forty-five pounds on his frame. He brought his concerns to a presenter at a marketing seminar who told him to seek me out and do my *Fat Loss After 40* program.

He contacted me, and we began a three-month journey. He dropped forty-five pounds and regained the full use of his body. Now, two years later, he is still at his chosen weight and whenever he gains unexpected weight—like during a cruise or vacation—he has the tools to get back down in a matter of days, not weeks or months.

This story can also be yours. It is very possible—you just have to follow the program.

While it is *simple*, it will not be easy.

I'm going to make an educated guess about why you might have picked up this book. In the past, whenever you put on a couple of pounds, you could work out a little harder, restrict your diet a bit, and get right back to your "ideal" weight (whatever that is).

However...

Ever since you hit thirty-five or forty *nothing seems to work!* You have tried everything—every pill, fad diet, and workout system. While some may provide short-term benefits, the weight *always* comes back with a vengeance, often bringing along pain and health issues.

At some point, you may have thought that it's time to "accept your age" and that you are no longer "young." As the pounds creep up on you, and you focus more on your business, career, or family, you rationalize that the days of being "fighting fit" or "fitting into that dress" are gone. But that is not the only problem. As ten pounds turns into twenty, then thirty, and so on, you start to wonder if you are shortening your life and worry about how this might mean leaving your children or your business a decade before your time. But how do you change that future?

You take the first step. Following the protocol in this book, I will teach you everything you need to change that future. In thirty days, you will be ten to fifteen pounds lighter, and I promise it will happen *without* starving yourself.

The *Fat Loss After 40* program will teach you how to:

- Prepare your mindset for success
- Follow an elimination diet to reduce inflammation and drop pounds
- Cleanse your liver of accumulated toxins to finally stop being fat
- Incorporate fasting into your program
- Use *one* exercise to boost Human Growth Hormone (HGH) and expedite fat loss
- Take supplements to optimize cellular energy
- Find the best way for you to work the program

The *Fat Loss After 40* program will also teach you NOT to:

- Do insane amounts of exercise—you are actually discouraged from working out for the first thirty days

- Starve yourself—you will control *what* you put in your mouth, but there is no caloric restriction, *ever*
- Waste thousands of dollars taking unnecessary or ineffective "weight loss" supplements—you will learn how to enhance cellular energy via readily available supplements, which are completely optional
- Expect to be "perfect"—people make mistakes, and you will learn how to recover from the occasional slip, so you can get back on track
- Worry about having to figure it out—the program is laid out for you
- Be overwhelmed—the program builds slowly

Why listen to me?

Because I know how to take men and women in their forties and beyond and effectively guide them to lose anywhere from ten to forty-five pounds and regain their health, vitality, and joy for life.

My name is Eric Guttmann, and I have written this book to share with you what I know. My *Fat Loss After 40* programs have helped people all over the world. I studied physical education in college and was a collegiate track and field athlete—a javelin thrower. I then joined and flew for the Navy, where I became a Certified Fitness Leader. I attended every course on physical training, healing, and nutrition on the outside that I could get my hands on and even started teaching seminars. In 2015, I started *Fat Loss After 40* online classes and seminars. Every year, I have kept on refining and improving them.

I have had many requests by clients, as well as those who have taken my workshops and seminars, to write this book, formalize my approach, and share the structure involved in a typical three-month *Fat Loss After 40* program.

Before we begin...

I am *not* a doctor.

I am *not* a nutritionist.

I am *not* talking about *any* medical condition; that is the realm of allopathic doctors, and *you* have to clear everything with your primary health care provider.

One last disclaimer: I know that red meat consumption can trigger some people, so if you find that you are not willing to eat it, then this program will not work for you.

If you have been struggling, keep reading and learn how to turn this around!

PART I

FIRST MONTH

CHAPTER 1

MINDSET AND THE CARNIVORE ELIMINATION DIET

MINDSET: HABITS VS. WILLPOWER

How much willpower do you burn on brushing your teeth? The answer should be little to none! Why? Because it's a habit that does not require willpower. You simply brush your teeth in the morning. You know what is *hard*? Trying not to eat cookies when you really want to eat cookies. That's called willpower and you will always lose out eventually because no one has unlimited amounts of willpower.

So how can we incorporate this into your *Fat Loss After 40* program? By adopting habits that make it easy. For example, if you don't turn on insulin in the morning (by eating sugary carbs) then it is a lot easier to control cravings. Eating nothing but protein and fat in the morning and turning it into a habit allows you to forgo the mental battle of sugar cravings and "struggling to eat right." Why? Because turning on insulin is a key hormonal (and therefore a battle you are bound to lose with willpower) indicator to deposit fat and crave more carbohydrates. With no insulin in the morning, then this hormonal loop is not activated and you simply go about your day without cravings instead of fighting them all day. Does that make sense?

The first two habits are the foundation that you will build your mindset on. You will set yourself up for success every day by doing two things each morning:

1. As soon as you wake up, get on the scale, and record your weight.

2. Text your weight to your accountability partner (someone you have chosen and trust to hold you to this morning practice).

The beauty about the daily text is that you know your actions will be tracked by someone who cares.

If you follow the program to the letter, you can drop anywhere from half a pound to two pounds every day! That is *if* you follow the program. Remember, the scale doesn't lie. As an accountability partner for my coaching clients, I've seen this sort of thing many times:

Monday: 260

Tuesday: 259

Wednesday: 258

Thursday: 257

Friday: 256

Saturday: 259 (and three hours late)

When this happens, I don't have to say anything, but I usually reply with, "Looks like somebody had a cheat day," and I leave it at that. No screaming. No scolding.

Building on the foundation of your mindset is the five-minute miracle practice which will really help you follow through on this program: decide your target goal weight and visualize hitting that target without losing sight of where you are starting from today. The human body and mind need a goal to focus on; this brings up energy and reserves not previously counted upon.

For example, one former naval officer had ballooned up to 265 pounds, and he needed to be at 230 pounds. The first thing I had him do was to get a 3 x 5 card and write: "By 1 Nov. 2021 I will weigh 230 pounds." Then I had him do this mental exercise every morning:

> Close your eyes and take a couple of deep breaths. Once you are calm remember what your bathroom looks like. Notice where the toilet, shower, and sink are and then imagine looking at yourself in your bathroom mirror.
>
> Now see yourself getting on the scale and seeing your target number. (In my friend's case, it was 230 pounds.) After looking down at the scale and seeing the number you are shooting for, look up at the mirror and see yourself as you want to be—flat stomach, abs showing, perhaps a vein running through the biceps, a square jaw, you get the idea. Get the feeling of accomplishment that achieving this weight will make you feel.
>
> By now, you should be smiling!
>
> Now, with your eyes still closed, change the image, and see yourself as you are right now—overweight, flabby, and with the actual number on the weight scale today. Now, imagine the desired end-state image on top and the reality image on the bottom at the same time.

Keeping a clear picture of where you are now compared to where you want to be might make you a little pissed off, which is good because it gets you to take *action!*

A critical component at this stage of the program is taking the time every morning to realize that all you have to do to achieve your target goal is establish a proper mindset (described above) and follow the steps described below. If you do that, the end result is as good as done!

REDUCE INFLAMMATION: THE CARNIVORE DIET

When you want to lose weight in your forties, you have to address things differently than when you were in your twenties. Gone are the days when you could just "work out a little more" and "eat a little less" to get quick results. For weight loss to be successful and sustainable, and before we even touch a weight or lace up a running shoe, we have to:

1. Reduce inflammation

2. Detoxify the liver

What happens if you don't address these things first? Well, most likely you will go overboard and injure yourself.

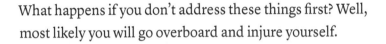

"Robert" had a SEAL-level of fitness in his youth and left the Navy to work a desk job for the government. In order to advance, he started working on his master's degree at night. During this period of time, he was sleeping about four hours a night and put on a lot of extra weight.

Once the Master's degree was over, he looked at himself and felt "disgusted" (men use that word a lot). He dug into his memory files and remembered exactly what he did when he was being trained by the US Navy SEALs.

He took his lunch hour to train and ruptured his liver; he had to go to the emergency room.

Now, most people do not have the mental toughness to push that hard, but this guy was no ordinary guy—he had been trained by the SEALs in his youth. Unfortunately, instead of starting where he actually was, he wanted to go back to his "in-his-prime" body.

A lot of men, upon being "disgusted" by what they see in the mirror, will take drastic actions by going into their past and getting "crazy." The only problem is that while you could do that in your twenties, your forty-year-old body is not going to put up with it. Why? Well, because you first need to reduce systemic and chronic inflammation.

How can you do this? By successfully completing a thirty-day Carnivore Experiment:

1. Follow a Carnivore Diet for thirty days.

2. Drink mostly water (you can drink black coffee or tea, but no soft drinks, alcohol, or adding sugar or creamer to coffee or tea).

That's it.

You may have questions like:

But, what about exercise?

Don't I need supplements?

Can I eat carbs? Eggs? Guacamole? Drink alcohol?

Stop and realize you *only* have to do *two* things for the next *two* weeks: eat meat and drink water. No negotiating.

This can work miracles for some, as you notice the pounds drop and the inflammation go away.

What do I mean by a Carnivore Diet?

1. Ideally, ribeyes and angus beef burgers. Any type of ruminant meat is preferable (beef, goat, deer, lamb, etc.), followed by poultry (chicken, turkey, etc.) and then followed by fish (salmon, tuna, sardines, etc.).

2. Bone broth, coconut oil, butter, water, and salt, as well as coffee and tea with no sugar or creamer, are also included.

One of my coaching clients had a total weight loss of twenty-five pounds in one month (without exercise). He bought a bunch of ribeyes and focused on ribeye steaks and angus beef burgers exclusively for thirty days. He did not "slip-up" even once, which is why he was so successful; a lot of people have multiple slip-ups, but even with those slip-ups, they still average ten pounds a month.

Upon beginning a Carnivore regimen I recommend you do the following:

1. **Feasting:** During the first three to five days, you are free to eat all the red meat you want as often as you want. The point is to actually begin feeding and absorbing fats

and proteins—perhaps for the first time. While it can be a "kid in the candy store" moment, the important thing is to eat to satiation.

2. **Intermittent Fasting (IF):** After three to five days of feasting, you'll move into a two-meals-a-day type program, which is frequently referred to as Intermittent Fasting (IF). Moving into a Carnivore IF program should be an effortless progression after your first three to five days of feasting. Most people end up skipping breakfast and ensuring they are properly hydrated while consuming black coffee with some form of healthy fat. This could be coconut oil, grass-fed butter, or medium chain triglycerides (MCT), which help to enhance the effects of caffeine by nourishing the brain without triggering digestion or spiking insulin. You can have your first solid food intake around 11:00 a.m. and your second meal at 5:00 p.m. This seems to be the norm with everyone, including myself. The idea is to have a sixteen-hour period where you are not ingesting solid food and an eight-hour feeding window where you eat all the calories of the day.

3. **One Meal a Day (OMAD):** After about two weeks on Carnivore IF, you can advance to a one-meal-a-day program (OMAD) for a couple of days out of the week, which is basically 23:1 IF (no solid food for twenty-three hours and a one-hour feeding window). During OMAD

there is absolutely no caloric restriction. If you feel like eating three or four ribeyes, then so be it. Even if you feel like eating five ribeyes—go for it! You will notice that you will eat the same amount of meat in pounds regardless of whether you eat two times a day or one time a day. For example, most men (on average) end up eating about two pounds of meat a day.

You may be wondering why this works. Let's pause for a second and think about all the stuff you will *not* be eating:

1. **Sugar:** if you are able to do this successfully, then it will mean that—perhaps for the *first* time in your life—you will go thirty days without sugar.

2. **Processed foods:** there is no defense for processed foods. Yes, they are convenient and inexpensive, but they lack any real nutrition and are literally "empty calories." To illustrate this point, a fellow naval officer I served with from the country of Uruguay once said to me (while stationed at Naval Station Mayport) that in his home country he can eat a small side of beef with vegetables, and he is full and satisfied. Yet in the US he can eat a burger and remain hungry and then eat a pizza. He asked me "why?" I let him know that it's because the food in his country is nutrient dense and the food here is nutrient deprived. His body still needed vitamins, minerals, and enzymes to work, and since he did not

get those from his first meal his body was telling him that he still needed to eat. To make matters worse, they are engineered to be addictive (you can't eat just one, huh?)—food companies hire scientists to make their products sweet, salty, and crunchy in the most addictive ways. Don't take my word for it. Google that shit!

3. **Vegetable oils:** the complete avoidance of vegetable oils for thirty days will have dramatic effects on inflammation. It took me a *long* time to realize that you could have the perfect organic diet, but if you cook it with highly inflammatory vegetable oils, your results will always be sidelined.

Let's review what I mean by Carnivore diet: meat, salt, water. The meat provides the fat and protein. The salt provides the minerals and flavor. Water, well, that one speaks for itself. Also, remember that during this thirty-day period, you can *only* use coconut oil or butter to cook your meat. Absolutely no corn, canola (whatever the hell that is), or any seed or vegetable oil.

One time while working at the Navy Yard I wanted to clean up my diet but was not doing Carnivore at the time. I consider myself a practical guy, so I went to the Asian food option on base and ordered the stir fry vegetables and teriyaki chicken without the sauce. That seems pretty clean, doesn't it?

Well, after three weeks of eating like this, my lower back pain got worse! My wife started asking questions, and I realized that it started getting worse when I started "eating clean." That's when I realized that the Achilles' Heel of most nutritional programs is oil. Even if you get organic meats and organic vegetables, if you cook them with vegetable oils, they become highly inflammatory!

When I do strict Carnivore, I usually lose ten pounds in the first week. How can that be? Well, it's taken me a while to accept this, but the reason must be *inflammation*.

I didn't drop ten pounds of fat in ten days. What left my body was the inflammation around tissues, which is why people who do Carnivore tend to improve three things: joint pain, gastrointestinal distress, and mental/anxiety issues.

You are probably wondering what results you can expect during your thirty-day Carnivore Experiment, in addition to the typical ten- to twenty-pound weight loss. Everyone's experience is different, but I'd like to share my thoughts from the first time I did a Carnivore Experiment.

CARNIVORE UPDATE: WEEK TWO

1. The last two days I have been a little tired; I guess at the two-week mark is where the rubber hits the road and where you really find out how addicted you are to food.

2. The interesting thing is that the foods that I want to

add when I am done with this experiment are Caesar salads, watermelons, and seasoned nuts (spicy nuts). I do *not* have any desire for starches or heavy processed sugars. I also had a vicious sweet tooth, and I am not craving any sugar.

3. This may sound counterintuitive, but eating this way makes you more "spiritual" and "conscious" about food. Cooking is a snap: warm skillet, butter, beef for one or two minutes, turn beef over for one or two minutes, eat. What you start to notice is that you are eating the body of an animal that had to give its life so that you may live. You don't get the same effect when your meat is disguised—for example, orange beef or a hamburger. I am much more grateful and a lot less "mindless" about my food.

4. I don't know what happens at the ten- to twelve-day mark, but I feel like I *completely* emptied my colon, and it feels great.

5. Sleep has been great this week, and I did not have to do any elaborate stretching and lacrosse ball rituals on my lower back to get there. Now I realize how much the sugar and starchy carbs (which turn to sugar once consumed) play a heavy role in triggering tightness and tension in my lower back.

6. I am noticing the difference between eating what your body needs versus eating out of boredom. Every now and then I get thoughts of, "*Oh it would be nice to taste this,*" but then I analyze what's going on, and I realize that these thoughts only happen when I am bored. Because I recognize this, I do not fall for the trap of eating crappy food. My body is well nourished, and I am not physically hungry; this allows me to resist these temptations.

7. One curious note is that when I take pre-workout supplements, they no longer have that "F@*k yeah! Let's train!" effect. Perhaps there is some relation between caffeine and carb consumption that spikes the feelings of energy. When I take them now, I am aware of them, and they are a nice "pick me up," but I remain much calmer.

8. My hair and nail growth are on steroids! Drinking one to two cups of bone broth a day and sucking the marrow out of bigger pieces, like beef shanks, has made my hair and nails grow at a much faster rate.

9. This week I started eating organ meats—specifically liver and kidney. The way I do this is to mix it in with ground beef so I can make hamburger patties that are 50 percent organ meat and 50 percent ground beef.

10. I haven't weighed myself, but my wife says I have lost some weight. That was not my goal at all, but I will check my weight at the end of thirty days to see where I am at.

CARNIVORE UPDATE: THIRTY DAYS

1. I increased my nutrient density—My first observation is that rather than looking at it through the lens of meat-only, it is best to look at it as an elimination diet where you remove everything except what is probably the most nutrient-dense food, which is meat (red meat, most of all).

2. I cut out harmful ingredients—Just like the vegans who say that perhaps the greatest benefit of the vegan diet in the first three months is not what you eat, but what you *don't eat*, perhaps the greatest benefit of the Carnivore Diet is what I was not eating: processed foods, sugar, food additives, chemicals, preservatives, MSG, etc.

3. My joint pain decreased considerably—I believe there is a direct link between sugary carb consumption and inflammation in the body. Reduce the inflammation in the body through diet and joint pain is minimized.

4. My sleep improved—perhaps due to the reason stated above, the reduction in inflammation and accompanying

joint pains meant that my sleep was not being interrupted by pain, tightness, and tension in my lower back.

5. I achieved emotional equanimity—the emotional rollercoaster is over, and I am rarely "hangry."

6. I lost weight—Yes, you drop weight effortlessly; I dropped ten pounds without really trying or "counting calories." I ate to satiation, which roughly meant two pounds of beef a day.

There's a logic behind this. The order in which food is digested in the body is: alcohol, carbs, fat, then protein.

OK, so a guy goes out for lunch and has a cheeseburger with fries and a beer. The body will not touch the carbs until it has completely digested all the beer. Let's say that in one hour the body digested all the beer. Fine, now it's moving towards the bread and the fries. So, let's say that in two hours the carbs are digested, and the body is ready to begin digesting the fat. Oh, but wait, it's been three hours since he last ate, and he gets himself a little snack—some chips, some sugary candy to give him a boost, you know the deal. Guess what—he reset the carb clock again. So two hours later, he digested the snack and is ready to digest the fat, but now he's home ready to start dinner.

Remember, the body has not fully digested and absorbed

the fat or proteins from lunch. Now he sits down and starts eating dinner. You guessed it! He reset the digestion process. This demonstrates why a lot of Americans never fully digest the fat and proteins that they consume.

Now, what happens when you eat the Carnivore Diet? According to this digestion model, there is no time wasted on alcohol and carbs, so the body goes straight to digesting fat. Fat you desperately need. Because you are satisfied for much longer and are not snacking in between, the full digestion cycle is able to be carried out and the fat and proteins you consume will be digested and assimilated. This can explain why people experience health benefits from the Carnivore Diet.

Before we move on, I'd like to highlight the benefit of breaking your addiction to sugar in all its forms during this thirty-day cycle, based on my own experience. It's very easy to consume sugar every day. We have been programmed to associate sugar with rewards and comfort.

One of the executive assistants at my work would place a dish with chocolates and sweets on her desk. A lot of us, including myself, would mosey on down to her area and get a couple of chocolates around 2–3 p.m. and have a nice chat.

And guess who got into a habit of eating three to five pieces of chocolate every day? That's right, this guy right here.

Now, I am an active person and have a predominantly healthy diet, so my thinking was that I could absorb the extra sugar and calories because I burn them through my lifestyle. I did not have any weight gain issues from the three to five pieces of chocolate, but I was probably having subsurface inflammation issues that I did not even notice. That is the insidious nature of this phenomenon.

What would be the effect of eating three to five pieces of chocolate every day for twenty years? Not good. The inflammation from sugar and carbs were affecting my body and were likely responsible for some of my lower back pain and sleeplessness at night. Both of which went down considerably when I stopped eating sugar.

Lastly, both myself and my son, who did this with me, experienced weight loss without restricting calories. I lost ten pounds, and my son lost a little more. While this weight loss was evenly distributed, it really helped in the midsection—so yes, I do have a flatter stomach and a smaller waist now. More importantly for my son, this experiment was able to eliminate gastro-intestinal discomfort that had been bothering him for years.

After completing thirty days of the Carnivore Diet, I began to reintroduce foods, beginning with a Caesar salad and strawberries, which I added to my evening steak.

They were delicious!

CHAPTER 2

HOMOZON AND SLEEP

HOMOZON

After two weeks on Carnivore, I invite you to try a product called Homozon, which was developed with the help of Nicola Tesla. While doing Carnivore you may end up having reduced bowel movements. At the two-week mark, you can get a product called Homozon which is a stool softener made of magnesium and ozone. When consumed internally, the ozone is liberated and the oxygen helps to clean out the colon in a healthy way.

Adding Homozon is not necessary for the program to be successful (it is completely optional), but if you are carrying around extra weight in the form of fecal matter—on top of fat—then this will help to clear it out. Once you finish your initial bag of Homozon, I recommend that you stop taking it and switch to taking magnesium-l-glycinate with your evening meal.

Magnesium is responsible for over 300 metabolic processes, and that is why when people supplement with magnesium-l-glycinate they report better sleep, lessened anxiety, better bowel movements, and in some cases, a reduction or elimination of muscle cramps.

The current estimate for magnesium-deficient people in the industrialized world is 88 percent. It is likely that you are one of them. There are tests to confirm, but look over the list of symptoms for magnesium deficiency and see if you have any: leg cramps, foot pain, muscle twitching, constipation, weakness, insomnia, numbness, tingles, personality changes (tense or anxious), abnormal heart rhythm, panic attacks, vertigo (fainting, dizziness, and falls), or high blood pressure.

If I had these symptoms, I would increase my magnesium intake, and my preferred form would be magnesium-l-glycinate. To be clear, you cannot get enough magnesium from the modern diet alone, and even with magnesium supplementation you could still be low.

SLEEP

An often overlooked factor that is crucial for fat loss and

health is sleep. For the longest time, I was sleeping five and a half hours a night. I would go to sleep around 11:30 p.m. and wake up at 5:00 a.m. While that was fine in my twenties and thirties, fueling my body with extra caffeine to make up the difference, I decided to fix that gap in my forties. (Also, as I got older, if I went to the bathroom at night, it would keep me awake for about an hour before I could go back to sleep.)

Now, I average seven to eight hours of sleep most nights, and it makes a huge difference. First of all, when you sleep eight hours, you are not craving sweets all of the time. When you don't get enough sleep, and your brain is tired, it wants to make up the difference with quick hits of sugar and caffeine. Once you start to sleep eight hours on a regular basis, it is a lot easier to do IF, and your emotional well-being improves.

When I started looking at my sleeping patterns, I noticed that there were two big culprits keeping me up at night—mental distractions and physical discomfort. The mental distractions could be overthinking or worry when I had a big or important task ahead of me. I would wake up at 3:00 a.m. and remember something I had forgotten to do for the next day. The physical discomfort was the one that got me most of the time—it was pain, tightness, and tension in my lower back! After addressing these two issues, sleep came much easier.

Below are my top ten tips for getting a good night's sleep:

1. **Avoid caffeine after 11:00 a.m.** The first and most obvious reason you may have trouble sleeping is over-consumption of caffeine. Many of my military peers would hit the gym at either their lunch break or at the end of the day. They would take their pre-workouts, and I noticed that the ones who took their pre-workouts later in the day would have the most trouble sleeping. Depending on your sensitivity, you may need to cut caffeine by 9:00 a.m. Others can drink a cup of coffee at night and go to sleep.

2. **Take 400 mg of magnesium-l-glycinate with dinner.** As I mentioned earlier, most of us in the western world are magnesium-deficient and need to supplement magnesium into our diet. Taking magnesium with your evening meal helps you to relax physically and mentally—a huge aid in getting a good night's sleep.

3. **Refrain from food and drink two to three hours before bedtime.** One of the reasons I was getting up to go to the bathroom was because I was always drinking water. Going to bed with a full stomach works against you getting a good night's sleep. Going two to three hours without food or drink prior to bedtime allows you to get a better night's sleep because your body will not be in the middle of digestion just as you want to sleep.

Additionally, if you are serious about improving your sleep, avoid alcohol at night as well (except on special occasions). Alcohol-induced sleep is not reparative.

4. **Walk for fifteen to thirty minutes after your dinner.** Most people spend the majority of their day sitting down. For a lot of folks, especially really busy ones over forty, making a habit of walking thirty minutes after dinner might be their only physical activity during most of the work week. Walking after dinner helps digestion, lubricates the joints, and serves as a physical, mental, and emotional tonic to release tension. Try it!

5. **Meditate.** The practice of meditation can help calm the mental chatter and allow you to relax better before sleep. Use whatever technique works for you.

6. **Write everything down before going to sleep.** One of the things that can keep you awake is trying to remember all the things you need to do. When I have a lot of things going on, I take a small notebook and write down all the things I am supposed to remember. This way I can dump it out of my mind and onto a page; my mind is freed from remembering all those details.

7. **Avoid screens for one to two hours before bed.** This can be part of a ritual where you either put a blue light filter on your devices or wear some blue light blocking

glasses. Ideally you should refrain from all artificial light before going to bed as that can alter your melatonin production, although a regular light bulb is OK if you are using it to read a fiction book to relax before going to bed instead of watching TV or cruising social media.

8. **Eliminate tightness and tension in your body.** Most nights I would fall asleep and ninety minutes later my lower back would wake me up. I would have to switch into a left-facing fetal position in order to release the pain and tension. I would eventually fall asleep, but ninety minutes later that tightness and tension would wake me up again. I would have to switch into a right-facing fetal position. That would purchase another ninety-minute cycle before the alarm went off. How did I fix it? By stretching the area at night and then using lacrosse balls on the tender points. Now, I stretch and use something called a Shakti Mat which I got for sixteen dollars on Amazon. It is supposed to mimic the "bed of nails" practice. I hold the mat for one-minute rounds on my lower back, and it seems to do the trick.

9. **Drink chamomile tea.** My wife turned me on to this, and while this does not work all the time, it works at least most of the time. Take it with your dinner or after your evening walk if you feel a little antsy or unable to go to sleep.

10. **Cleanse your liver.** This is coming up in the next chapter, but it's worth mentioning the Liver Cleanse here because it tends to improve everyone's sleep. Liver cleansing is something you can do in a day and a half, and you will notice that sleep improves right after you do it.

Of course, the main drivers to a good night's sleep are a healthy diet and a regular exercise program as opposed to a "quick fix" solution.

On the *Fat Loss After 40* program, most people start having better sleep after going Carnivore, releasing the lower back, and taking magnesium-l-glycinate. When people finish the Liver Cleanse at the end of their first thirty days on the program, their sleep dramatically improves.

> If you snore, you should have a sleep study done to see if you qualify for a Continuous Positive Airway Pressure (CPAP) machine. This is a discussion you need to have with your doctor. Many of my military friends who have been put on CPAP report improvement in their sleep. You may also want to get a full checkup with your doctor to ensure that there are no hormonal or endocrine reasons affecting your sleep.

Do you want to learn how to do the Liver Cleanse?

Read on, and I will tell you all about it!

CHAPTER 3

LIVER CLEANSE

After age forty, the liver is the bottleneck to fat loss. In our twenties, the liver operates efficiently, despite all the drinking and excess of our youth. That is why you can go out drinking in your twenties until 2:00 a.m., sleep for four hours, wake up at 6:00 a.m., hit the gym, and carry on with the rest of the day like nothing happened. In your forties, that is *not* the case. If I were to drink more than two glasses of wine at a formal event, then I would have to take two days off from training.

The comment I hear most is, "Eric, I have tried everything to lose weight! I have counted calories and starved myself while exercising like a madman (or madwoman) and *nothing* seems to work. Help!"

The liver is one the body's main detoxifiers. For our purposes, consider anything that the body cannot utilize as a nutrient to be a toxin. This includes substances from alcohol, pharmaceutical drugs, and recreational drugs to food additives, preservatives, food coloring, and building materials (asbestos). Even oil and gas (remember how you liked the smell of gas as a kid), jet fuel (I flew in the Navy and inhaled plenty of JP-5 and JP-8, which is jet fuel), and the myriad of new chemicals our bodies are exposed to on a yearly basis are toxins. When there are more toxins than your liver can safely clear, it encapsulates them in fat, preventing those toxins from getting into your bloodstream.

A lot of the fat that people over forty carry is not just "extra calories," but encapsulated toxins that the body has been storing since childhood, and the liver never got a chance to clear.

Stop for one minute.

If you have previously tried and failed at weight loss, and you did so without incorporating the liver, then you have to realize that it's *not* your fault!

SMART TARGETING THE LIVER

Did you know that a lot of bodybuilders have scarred livers similar to that of raging alcoholics? No, it's not the anabolic steroids. Traditional bodybuilding has a person bulking upwards of fifty pounds in the "off-season," in a combination of fat and muscle, and then shredding them in the three months prior to the competition. The real cause of the damage is dropping all that fat in such a short time with all those encapsulated toxins hitting the liver at a rate greater than it can safely detoxify. It is important to detoxify carefully.

Bombing runs in World War II were called carpet bombing (completely covering an area)—to hit one German factory they would literally bomb the whole city, leading to a lot of collateral damage. Today, we use smart weapons to ensure that we hit the exact target while minimizing collateral damage.

Most traditional liver cleansing products are like carpet bombs—aimed at your body.

You can drink dandelion tea and buy all sorts of "liver care" pills and tablets and still not get the results that you will get in a day and a half from my targeted Liver Cleanse.

Not only are the results significant, but the actual components of the Liver Cleanse are easily accessible to you: distilled water, Epsom salts, organic olive oil, organic grapefruit, organic green apples, and Himalayan salt. The cost per cleanse should amount to no more than $20, and a lot of the components will last you one to two years.

LIVER CLEANSE IN LAYMAN'S TERMS

Before getting technical (I provide specific directions for the Liver Cleanse at the end of this chapter), let me just explain what the Liver Cleanse is. First, there is a lot of excitement and curiosity at the prospect of dropping five to eight pounds in a day and a half, but sometimes there is a little resistance. So, let me try to assuage your concerns by explaining it in layman's terms.

Your gallbladder stores a certain amount of bile based on how much fat you consume. Your body has a "cellular memory" of approximately how much bile your body needs to produce to deal with your typical meals. Let's say, for the sake of argument, that your body produces ten units of bile for your standard breakfast. Ok, but you will not eat any breakfast or anything with protein or fat for that matter. "No problem," your body says, "I will just save it and dump it at lunch." Then lunch hour comes along, and you do not eat lunch or anything with protein or fat. Again, for the sake of argument, let's say your body produces twenty units of bile to deal with lunch. "No problem," your body says, "I will just save it and dump it at dinner." Then dinner time rolls around, and lo and behold, you had no dinner or anything with fat and/or protein. Let's assume that dinner is the heaviest meal of the day for you and that your body is used to producing thirty units of bile to deal with your dinner. Now your gallbladder and liver are "all dressed up to go to the dance" with nowhere to go.

Then what do you do at 9:30 p.m.? You drink one cup of organic olive oil. (Don't worry, I will explain the full process a little later on.) And what do you think happens to your liver and gallbladder when you do this? Well, it's like a zit or pimple that is ready to burst and you pinch it and all the contents in the proximal end "burst" into the colon, and the next day you end up feeling like a million bucks, along with dropping anywhere from five to eight pounds.

LIVER CLEANSE ORIGINS

In the 1990s, a nurse by the name of Hulda Clarke came out with a book called *The Cure for All Disease* in which she explained how completely clearing the liver could help the body heal from all conditions.

There are miles of bile ducts (50,000 by some estimates) in the liver. When your body encounters a toxic substance, the body protects you by encapsulating it in fat, mucus secretions, or fatty accumulations in the liver. When you overburden your liver with more toxic material than it can process, then you create a toxic situation within your body. A lot of degenerative diseases are attributed to this systemic accumulation of toxic material over a lifetime.

When you perform the Liver Cleanse, you will remove "waxy pellets." These are made of cholesterol, which is manufactured in the liver. Eighty percent of the cholesterol in the body is produced in the liver. Ninety-five percent of these pellets are waxy agglomerations of coagulated cholesterol. These cholesterol "pellets" clog the bile ducts in the liver and the gallbladder.

Sometimes bile ducts are full of cholesterol crystals that did not form into "pellets." They appear as "chaff" and clearing this chaff is just as important as purging pellets. Most people will need to clear a total of 2,000-3,000 pellets before their livers are clear enough to be rid of allergies, bursitis, and upper back pain.

Let's get something clear, these "pellets" are not stones in the medical sense. What we are talking about are simply the waxy cholesterol pellets that tend to block the ducts. These are soft, pliable, and will *not* show up on an X-ray. When someone is told that they have stones, it means a calcification that will show up on an X-ray. Those stones require surgery, and that's not what we are talking about; so, rest assured that this will not be a painful or complicated process.

How do you know the difference between these "pellets" and feces?

Very simple, when you poop (and, after taking the Epsom salts, you will), look in the toilet. All the feces will sink to the bottom and be brown. The "pellets" will be white, green, or yellowish and will float to the top (because they are made of fat). What I do is count the number of pellets floating (or make an approximation). Sometimes, you also release a lot of chaff, which looks like, well, chaff—small, yellowish, and sand-like.

Some say it takes about ten liver cleanses for the liver to be "finally clean." Others have overcome "incurable" diseases like multiple sclerosis and Crohn's disease by doing one liver cleanse a month for eighteen months.

When you do two consecutive liver cleanses, and no pellets come out, then your liver is considered clean.

BENEFITS OF THE LIVER CLEANSE

1. The forty-two- to forty-eight-hour fast provides a period of rest that allows the body to heal.

2. The liver and gallbladder flush is one of the main reasons people do the Liver Cleanse. I pass from 120-200 pellets per Liver Cleanse. During my fourth Liver Cleanse, I passed a white mass the size of a thumb. During another Liver Cleanse, I passed seven large apricot-kernel-sized masses.

3. As a bonus, the colon is also cleansed (thanks to the Epsom salts) because in order for the liver and gallbladder to flush, the colon needs to be emptied.

4. This particular Liver Cleanse also re-mineralizes and tops off your magnesium. We already discussed how important magnesium is—responsible for over 300 metabolic processes—and that it is a mineral in which most people in the Western world are deficient, resulting in many health issues.

5. I include Himalayan salt because most of us are deficient in minerals due to the low mineral content of the soil. When you give the body the basic building blocks it needs, aka minerals, it can perform properly.

6. Many experience more energy and increased endurance. In my case, I increased my jump rope circuit from fifteen to thirty rounds.

7. Because your body is performing better, the recovery time after exercise is faster.

8. The absorption of food and supplements improves because the colon has been emptied, and the liver and gallbladder have been flushed.

9. Weight Loss. Every time I do the Liver Cleanse, I drop five or six pounds; others have dropped up to eight pounds from a single Liver Cleanse.

10. For some reason I can't fully explain, the skin gets a noticeable glow after the Liver Cleanse.

11. Chinese medicine states the state of the liver is reflected in the eyes. The day after the Liver Cleanse, the eyes are whiter and brighter.

12. Also in Chinese medicine, it is believed that the liver stores anger; perhaps the Liver Cleanse helps to flush out "emotional toxins" because there are many reports of feeling emotionally well and calm afterward.

13. Perhaps as a result of emotional well-being, many feel an increase in appreciation for family members.

14. When you forgo the pleasure of eating for forty-two to forty-eight hours, you develop your willpower and self-confidence. Look at it as weightlifting for your will.

15. Some (including me) do the Liver Cleanse with no caffeine or supplements, which is a great way to challenge your addictions. (Optional: I now do the Liver Cleanse with guarana tablets to avoid caffeine withdrawal.)

16. If you meditate or do qigong, you will find that your energy and sensitivity increases after the Liver Cleanse. Your mind is sharp, and your energy follows your will. Intuition also improves.

17. It feels as if your internal organs were a dirty windshield, and you took a squeegee and removed all the caked-on dirt and left it clear and shiny. Your internal organs feel clear and light, and it is easier to smile!

18. The Liver Cleanse makes allergies go away or greatly diminish. (Raw local honey and bee pollen also help tremendously!)

19. I have routinely noticed that after a liver cleanse, libido improves. Also, you may start getting "wood" at 3 a.m., and as we know, "wood" is the poor man's testosterone test.

20. In addition to all of these benefits, there have been reports that the Liver Cleanse helps with psoriasis (one person reported as much as a 75 percent reduction in her psoriasis after just one Liver Cleanse), fibromyalgia, osteoarthritis, rheumatoid arthritis, lower back pain, irritable bowel syndrome (IBS), Crohn's disease, premenstrual syndrome (PMS), prostate problems, diabetes, multiple sclerosis, and cancer.

OK, would you like to know how to do it? Great! Let's get to work.

ERIC GUTTMAN LIVER PROTOCOL 5.0

THREE DAYS BEFORE THE CLEANSE

Leading up to your Liver Cleanse, spend three days drinking ½ gallon of distilled water for every one hundred pounds of body weight each day. If you work out, add another ½ gallon.

The preferred method for drinking distilled water is one to two glasses thirty minutes before eating and another one to two glasses ninety minutes after eating. Upon awakening, drink one to two glasses on an empty stomach—this step is important to prevent nausea during the Liver Cleanse due to dehydration.

Optional: drink one cup of organic apple juice with your last meal of the day for seven days prior to your Liver Cleanse.

Day 1

When following the schedule below, prepare three glasses of hot, distilled water and Epsom salt in the morning; you want the Epsom salts to be fully dissolved when you drink them in the evening (and the next morning).

It's also important to note that your organic green apple juice must come from at least four green apples. Putting the green apples through a juicer and drinking the juice immediately is best. Juice from organic red apples is second best; bottled, organic store-bought juice is a distant third (flash pasteurized if possible). *Do not use commercial apple juice* (it's nothing but sugar water).

8:00 a.m.	Drink 16 oz. distilled water with ½ teaspoon of Himalayan Salt
8:30 a.m.	Drink 16 oz. distilled water with ½ teaspoon of Himalayan salt
9:30 a.m.	Drink one glass of organic green apple juice
10:30 a.m.	Drink 16 oz. distilled water with ½ teaspoon of Himalayan salt
11:30 a.m.	Drink 16 oz. distilled water with ½ teaspoon of Himalayan salt
1:30 p.m.	Drink one glass of organic green apple juice
2:00 p.m.	Do not eat or drink anything other than what is outlined in this Liver Cleanse after 2:00 p.m.
6:00 p.m.	Drink one cup of water with two tablespoons of Epsom salt
8:00 p.m.	Drink one cup of water with two tablespoons of Epsom salt
9:30 p.m.	Drink one cup of organic olive oil and one cup of organic grapefruit juice (mixed together)

After drinking your organic olive oil and grapefruit juice, lay down and stay still for twenty minutes; you may move after twenty minutes have passed.

Day 2

When following the schedule below, make sure you drink the third glass of Epsom salt drink upon awakening.

8:00 a.m.	Drink one cup of water with two tablespoons of Epsom salt
9:00 a.m.	Drink one cup of distilled water
9:30 a.m.	Drink one cup of distilled water
10:00 a.m.	Drink one cup of distilled water
10:30 a.m.	Drink one cup of distilled water
11:00 a.m.	Drink one cup of distilled water
11:30 a.m.	Done

After finishing the Liver Cleanse, you may eat lunch. I also suggest taking a warm or hot bath with Epsom salts.

Be sure to count the pellets when you're finished.

Now, go and look at your calendar and schedule a day and a half when you can relax at home and complete your Liver Cleanse.

PART II

SECOND MONTH

CHAPTER 4

SLO-MO BEGINNER WORKOUT

After your first month, you should have dropped anywhere from ten to fifteen pounds, reduced inflammation, improved your gut health, and performed a liver cleanse.

Now, you are ready to start adding some form of physical exercise.

Considering the average participant of *Fat Loss After 40* is about forty-five years old, has put on thirty to forty-five pounds that they want to drop, and may not have engaged in any form of physical exercise in months or years, we need to begin with the safest and most effective form of exercise.

SLO-MO WORKOUTS

Slow-motion (slo-mo) bodyweight exercise has been my tried and true method for working with people in the *Fat Loss After 40* program in the first month. After that, they graduate to more dynamic exercises, but for now, let's explain why slo-mo is best at this point.

Slo-mo exercises have the double benefit of being super safe by moving at a very slow speed through the *full* range of motion and extremely effective because you maximize the time under tension (TUT).

SLO-MO SQUAT

Set a timer for two minutes.

From a standing position start squatting down (if you need to hold onto something for balance, that's OK) at a pace of ten seconds to get from top to bottom.

Without pausing, as soon as you hit the bottom of the squat, begin standing up from the squat at a rate of ten seconds to get from the bottom to the top.

One squat equals twenty seconds of TUT.

If done properly, a two-minute round will have you performing six squats.

Instead of increasing weight or reps to improve, here you keep the time constant and look to minimize the reps by making each rep longer.

Talk to me when you can do *one* squat in two minutes! That's right—take one minute from top to bottom and one minute from the bottom back to the top.

This gives you clear guidelines for improvement and helps to remove the desire to jack up the weight or do more reps than your body can handle.

For your first month, do three rounds of slo-mo squats at two minutes on/two minutes rest.

SLO-MO PUSH-UP

Follow this with three rounds of Slo-mo Push-ups at the interval of one minute on/one minute rest.

In the case of the push-up, begin with the intention of taking five seconds to go from top to bottom and another five seconds to go from the bottom to top.

This means that if you can hold that pace, you would do six reps per minute.

If you want to improve, elongate the "travel" time from

five seconds to ten seconds; this would mean doing three reps per minute.

SLO-MO BICYCLE CRUNCH

The third exercise will be the Slo-mo Bicycle Crunch.

Lie on your back and slowly bring one knee up while bringing your opposite elbow to touch it—as you slowly extend that leg, start bringing the other knee up to meet with the other elbow.

Aim for twelve to sixteen reps per one-minute round, and do three rounds of one-minute exercise/one-minute rest.

For the fourth exercise, I am going to give you an option: the Easy Burpee or the Vacuum.

If you have any issues that prevent you from doing the Easy Burpee, then I recommend you finish with the Vacuum exercise.

EASY BURPEE

The key to this exercise is to go at your own pace and to perform each movement with the breath pattern indicated. Since you are going to be working in one-minute rounds, do not worry about the number of reps.

If you only get five clean reps, then that is all you need; eventually, your numbers will increase.

If, on the other hand, you are free of any aches, pains, or injuries that allow you to move at a faster clip in good form, then go for it.

The purpose of this exercise at the end is to tie all the movements of the body into one dynamic motion.

Also, it puts you in a good mood.

Without further ado, here is how to do it:

- Start from a regular standing position.
- Inhale as you bend your knees into a tucked position and place your hands on the ground.
- Exhale as you explode your legs out into a plank position.
- Inhale as you bring your legs back to the tucked position.
- Exhale as you spring into the standing position.

A technique that helps is calling this the "four-count burpee," where you forcefully say the number of the move you are executing:

- After you inhale and bend your knees into a tucked position, say, "One!"

- When you exhale and kick your legs out and arrive at the plank, "Two!"
- When you inhale and return to the tucked position, "Three!"
- And, finally, when you stand, "Four!"

This forceful calling out of the numbers tends to give you an extra *oomph* to commit to the exercise and seems to build the determination to finish it.

Aim for three rounds of one-minute exercise followed by a one-minute rest.

If you are unable (or unwilling) to do the Easy Burpee, then I suggest you finish with the Vacuum.

VACUUM

Remember the old-school bodybuilders?

They all had small waists even though they had bulging muscles.

Do you know why?

Because they believed in practicing the Vacuum exercise to keep their waists slim. Yes, they did anabolic steroids, but they did not use Human Growth Hormone (HGH).

Do you know why small waists fell out of favor?

The advent of artificial HGH in the bodybuilding world around the 1990s–2000s led to extended bellies becoming the norm due to enlarged organs, which made the practice of the Vacuum irrelevant.

The vacuum exercise is still practiced in yoga and other "physical culture" practices.

Here is how I recommend you do it:

- Begin with a bent-over position, hands on your knees.
- Take a deep breath to the point where your abdomen bulges out.
- Slowly exhale all the air from your lungs.
- Once all the air is out of the lungs, start pulling your stomach in; visualize trying to get the belly button to touch the spine.
- You are still in the bent-over position. Once you have achieved the deepest vacuum you can hold (belly button to lumbar vertebrae) slowly start standing up while holding the vacuum and bringing your hands from your knees to behind your ears.
- Hold for three to five seconds.

Recover from this exercise by doing deep inhales and exhales.

I recommend starting with six "reps" of this exercise; however, go up to ten if you feel good.

Standing up completely erect while holding the Vacuum is more than just for the show. What you are doing is elongating the trunk while in the fully vacuumed position to gently compress and tonify the internal organs.

CHAPTER 5

FASTING 24-48-72

After your first month on the *Fat Loss After 40* program, you will have lost about ten to fifteen pounds, been sugar free for thirty days, and have performed one liver cleanse. That's a lot for one month and serves to build a foundation for your second month where we start to add physical exercise. One of the other strategies that we start to incorporate in the second month is fasting.

Yes, *fasting!*

Fasting means refraining from food and drinking only water. Dry fasting means to refrain from food *and* water. Fasting is a way to train your body and mind because you are refraining from eating, and trust me, you will want to eat. After your first month, you will be comfortable with IF and even OMAD, so doing a twenty-four-hour fast is not such a big stretch.

I recommend you follow the Gracie Diet approach to fasting, which advocates going a twenty-four-hour period without food by skipping dinner one day and breakfast the next day. For example, on Friday, eat your lunch at 12:00 p.m., skip dinner, go to sleep, and sleep in late (if you can), skip breakfast, and then eat lunch again Saturday at 12:00 p.m. Voila! There's a twenty-four-hour fast.

A twenty-four-hour fast will reset your body, help you drop weight faster, and train your mind. One of the benefits of fasting versus caloric restriction is that fasting will boost your testosterone and growth hormone while caloric restriction will make you feel weak and lethargic. People do not lose muscle when fasting but waste away in caloric restriction.

Although people have been able to triumph over significant health challenges with fasting, you are simply focusing on giving your system a rest to help expedite fat loss after forty.

One big key to water fasting is to add minerals to your water. I recommend you look up the Snake Juice recipe on YouTube and either make a mineral blend of your own or simply purchase one of the options available. After you are able to successfully do a twenty-four-hour fast, wait a couple of weeks and work your way up incrementally to a forty-eight-hour fast. You do *not* have to jump straight into a forty-eight-hour fast. You can look at scheduling a thirty-hour fast.

However...

Here is an interesting tidbit—a thirty-hour fast means that you have lunch one day and then skip breakfast and lunch the next day and eat again at dinner. Everyone, myself included, does the mental math and realizes that if we just skipped dinner and went to sleep, we could have a forty-two-hour fast under our belt when we eat breakfast the next day. And if you have already trained yourself not to eat breakfast in the morning, then skipping breakfast and holding out to lunch will give you a forty-eight-hour fast.

There is no set schedule or urgency to get to the forty-eight- and seventy-two-hour fast mark, but there is the intention to do them within the time that is right for you. It will be quite a mental accomplishment when you knock out a twenty-four-, forty-eight-, and then a seventy-two-hour fast.

Once you realize that a twenty-four-hour fast is nothing, then you can work on scheduling longer fasts. And if you ever have a crazy weekend and put on eight pounds you know you have two tools to get you back on track: liver cleansing and fasting.

If you do nothing more than get in the habit of doing one twenty-four-hour fast a month along with IF, that alone will pay you *huge* dividends in your health and fat loss goals.

PART III

THIRD
MONTH

CHAPTER 6

UPHILL SPRINTS TO BOOST HGH

There is one exercise that can help you melt fat like a blow-torch, boost Human Growth Hormone (HGH), help release negative emotions (like fear, worry, and anxiety), increase your productivity to tackle "hard" tasks, and raise your libido. It is also the most effective exercise you can do to drop weight. It's Uphill Sprints.

THE BENEFITS AND DRAWBACKS OF HGH

HGH injections have been touted as a veritable fountain of youth in anti-aging circles. Claims of skin tightening, increased performance, reduced body fat, feeling and looking ten years younger, along with improved libido and sexual performance entice many affluent persons to give this a try. I say affluent because the cost runs from $1,500 to $2,000 a month for HGH injections, which require meticulous doses and daily injections.

HGH injections also have negative side effects, such as enlarged organs. If you notice a bodybuilder with that Cro-Magnon look, that indicates an overuse of HGH because their foreheads enlarge, and their bellies are distended from the internal organs growing bigger and pushing out.

The good news is that Uphill Sprints produce HGH naturally, for free, and they don't have the negative side effects like enlarged organs.

UPHILL SPRINTS HELP TO CLEAR OUT NEGATIVE EMOTIONS

Let's face it, 2020 and 2021 were tough on a lot of people. In my personal case this was compounded by the fact that I was leaving the military and had to start a whole new life. I had to decide between leaving Virginia and a guaranteed six-figure job in the government and moving to Florida to start from scratch. I have a wife and four kids to feed, so if you think that wasn't stressful then you're mistaken. Even though my wife and I had decided it was time to leave the Navy, which was like an "amicable divorce" where both parties can still "be friends," I faced a lot of doubt and uncertainty. The bottom line is that both my wife and I had a slew of worries affecting us on a daily basis.

Our saving grace was that we had a public park within ten minutes walking distance from our home. While I originally started doing the uphill sprints with my wife because her gym was closed, and she was looking for ways to stay active, we immediately noticed that on the days we did uphill sprints, a lot of the emotional stuff would disappear (for that day).

I have a theory that the "huffing and puffing" required for the sprinting effort helps to clear negative emotions from the internal organs. In Chinese medicine it is stated that certain emotions can negatively affect certain organs. For example, grief and sadness is said to affect the lungs; anger, frustration, and irritability impact the liver; fear, the kidneys; worry, the spleen; despair and lack of enthusiasm, the heart.

Well, to be honest, between my wife and I, we were probably feeling all of them! We both noticed that on the days we did uphill sprints, all of these negative emotions, worries, and preoccupations just seemed to melt away. While the "problems" were still there, we were now smiling with a "second wind."

Which leads to my next observation...

UPHILL SPRINTS IGNITE PRODUCTIVITY TO TACKLE DISTASTEFUL TASKS

My wife and I both noticed that on the days we did uphill sprints, our ability to knock out all distasteful tasks suddenly increased. My theory is that once you complete an uphill sprint workout, especially in the morning, then that was the "hardest" thing for the day, and everything else becomes easier by comparison. The liberation of negative emotions provides you with something of a "clean slate."

But I also noticed that, on the evenings we did Uphill Sprints...

LIBIDO INCREASED

Both my wife and I have an increase in libido and an increase in performance on our uphill sprints days. This has also been the experience of my clients, and it can be your experience as well.

UPHILL SPRINTS REDUCED RISK OF INJURY

Why uphill sprints and not regular flat sprints? The incline serves as a safety factor. By increasing the torque required to go forward, you minimize the chance of pulling a muscle.

I used to be a collegiate javelin thrower, and I would do my general physical preparation with the sprinters. My track and field coach explained to me that when people are training, they are either training their aerobic system or their anaerobic system to be efficient. He said, "That's why the hardest events to coach are the ones that are located in the middle of the anaerobic and aerobic threshold, like 800-meter hurdles." He explained that because I was a javelin thrower, "You are training your anaerobic system to be great. Therefore, you should never run more than six continuous miles in your training as that would decrease your performance as a javelin thrower." I loved training with the sprinters!

When I joined the Navy, I kept a penchant for sprints, and one day while I was stationed at Naval Station Mayport in Florida, I took my lunch hour to sprint. Because I had become much stronger through weightlifting, and my legs were bigger and more powerful than when I was a collegiate athlete, I actually pulled a muscle while sprinting on flat ground. I had to stop immediately, and that set me back a couple of weeks.

As I started getting into strongman training: steel bending, phone book tearing, and card tearing, I remember reading a book that stated that uphill sprints were safer for the body and minimized the chance of injury. Ever since I switched to uphill sprints, I have *never* pulled a muscle while sprinting.

IDEAL SPRINT DISTANCE

You might be surprised that I recommend the uphill sprint distance to be about forty to sixty meters or 120–180 feet. This is because humans naturally start decelerating after forty meters.

If the "rule" for stimulating your body to produce testosterone could be simplified to "lift heavy things," then the rule for HGH could be simplified to do things that make you "huff and puff." Yeah, I know, not exactly scientific explanations, but I can tell you from personal experience that these explanations, as rudimentary as they are, have proven to be true.

Here is how I do it (remember sprint distances are roughly forty to sixty meters):

Begin with a thorough joint mobility warmup. Activate the glutes with a "glute walk"—simply walk up the hill swinging your arms and ensuring that the glutes get turned with every step. If you need to, you can put your hands on your butt to ensure they are contracting with every upward step.

Your first sprint will start slow; you should only give ten to twenty percent effort. With each set, you will increase your effort.

Do not go 100 percent in your first set, ever!

Remember to rest for two minutes between sets one, two, and three. Rest for three to four minutes between sets four, five, and six.

SET	SPEED	
Warmup	Uphill walk (five minutes)	Engage your glutes with each step.
1	10-20 percent	Do as much as your body is willing at this speed.
2	20-30 percent	Do as much as your body is willing at this speed.
3	30-40 percent	Your body should start priming now.
4	50 percent (or more)	Your body should feel like going faster; do not run faster than your capability.
5	60 percent (or more)	You will notice the ability to run faster; listen to your body and let it do what it wants to do.
6	As fast as you dare	This should be the culmination of what your body can do that day.
Cooldown	Walk (five minutes)	Evaluate how you feel.

If you feel good after the sixth sprint, you may add another sprint. If after the seventh sprint, you feel good and want to do another one, then you may do an eighth sprint.

Do not do more than eight sprints!

NUTRITIONAL RECOMMENDATIONS FOR SPRINT WORKOUTS

I like to do this in the morning, preferably in a fasted state. I will have some form of caffeine, and 5 grams of L-glutamine prior to my workout. L-glutamine has been shown to help increase HGH production when paired with uphill sprints. I also mix another 5 grams of L-glutamine with water after my workout.

The most important thing to avoid shutting down your HGH production is to refrain from eating sugar and carbs immediately after your sprint workout. Wait thirty to sixty minutes before eating to allow your post exercise HGH to peak as much as it can.

As a general rule, when I do my sprints in the morning, I have my first solid food intake around 11:00 a.m., and it is usually a fat/protein meal with no carbs. For example, eggs and sausage.

You do *not* need to sprint to incorporate the principles in this chapter.

I would like to end this chapter with a very important point. I want you to focus on the *principles* in this chapter. What this means is that if you have some kind of condition that prevents you from running, whether it be plantar fasciitis, lower back pain, knee pain, hip pain, or any other ailment, *or* if you simply can't find a small incline where you live, you can still follow the protocol in any medium that is safe and effective for you to do.

This may include swimming, treadmill, exercise bike, stepper, elliptical, rowing, bicycle, versa climber, battling ropes, upper body ergometer, or even just walking steeper inclines at slower speeds.

Finally, one word of caution. I encourage you to work with your body—you must run *your race* and not anyone else's. If you are using a treadmill, it is always tempting to increase the speed and the incline to levels that are beyond your capacity. When this happens then you are courting injury. If you leave a workout in pain then you are not going to want to do it again, and the key to this whole *Fat Loss After 40* can be summarized in one word: *consistency*.

You might not believe me until you actually do it, but when I sprint in the "real" world, my knees and lower back feel great! Yes, that's right—my body will actually feel great and pain subsides when I work out at *my* proper levels in the real world as opposed to machines.

With that said, let me share one of my mistakes. My two oldest sons aged twenty and eighteen have actually blossomed into young men. The last time I went sprinting with my wife and second son, who has become somewhat of a fitness buff, I let him go first with the idea that I would catch up to him—as I always did. Well, just as I was starting to match my son's pace, I felt my lower back and hip kick into pain, so I immediately went back to running *my race* and let my son win. I am proud of him for finally surpassing me. I hope this will drive home the point of why you need to run *your race*.

I can't wait to hear your stories of success with Uphill Sprints or whatever modality you choose to implement. Just remember that if you are "huffing and puffing" then you did it right, no need to overthink it!

CHAPTER 7

ANTI-AGING STACKS AND SUPPLEMENTS

Note: I am not a doctor or a nutritionist. I am telling you what I do. I am not recommending you take anything. I encourage you to do your own research and make your own decisions.

VITAMIN D

Get some sun! If you have access to the sun, try to get fifteen minutes of exposure or more a day. If you do not have access to the sun, vitamin D supplements can help. I take 5,000 IU for every one hundred pounds of body weight when I don't have access to the sun. This means that for two months a year I take 10,000 IU and pair it with a vitamin K supplement to aid in absorption. The rest of the time I walk on the beach to get my vitamin D through natural sun exposure.

As a side note, fifteen to thirty minutes of sun exposure that does not burn, but turns the skin slightly red, is associated with the body producing 20,000 IU of vitamin D.

OMEGA-3 / L-CARNITINE / COQ10

This is both an anti-aging stack and a fat loss stack that can help you lose a couple of pounds and increase cellular energy.

This is the way it was explained to me:

The omega-3 helps to mobilize fat, the L-carnitine helps to transport the fat into the cells, and the CoQ10 turns on the mitochondria to use that fat for cellular energy.

I like to take 2 grams of omega-3, 1 gram of L-carnitine, and 200–400 mg of CoQ10 with a meal. When looking at omega-3 supplements, look at the eicosapentaenoic acid (EPA) and docosahexaenoic acid (DHA) numbers. EPA is good for the heart and DHA is good for the brain.

In regards to L-carnitine look for "Carnipure" on the back of the supplement bottle. The brand itself is secondary to ensuring you have Carnipure as the source of L-carnitine.

When it comes to CoQ10, if you are over forty, use the reduced form of CoQ10, which is called ubiquinol. Conventional CoQ10 is known as ubiquinone and up to your thirties, your body can take this and convert it into ubiquinol which is 70 percent more absorbable than ubiquinone. After your thirties, your ability to convert CoQ10 into ubiquinol goes down, thus taking the reduced form is recommended when you are over forty. More important than the brand is the source; I only consume Kaneka ubiquinol, which you can find on the back of the supplement bottle.

When I lived in El Salvador and had access to fresh fish, I did not consume omega-3 supplements. By fresh fish, I mean that the fish were swimming in the water that morning, were brought to my home at 11:00 a.m., and I was eating them for dinner at 5:00 p.m. The fish was so fresh that it did not smell or have a "fishy" taste—the only flavoring required was butter. If you also consume fresh fish on a regular basis, you may opt out of the omega-3.

If cost becomes an issue, you can forgo the L-carnitine or just do it every couple of months. When it comes to ubiquinol I am on it year round. This is the only supplement that I consider a *must* for people over forty, and I take 200 mg or more *daily*. If I was independently wealthy, I would be on 400 mg or more of ubiquinol year-round.

MAGNESIUM-L-GLYCINATE

I have 400 mg of magnesium-l-glycinate with dinner and find that it helps me to relax at the end of the day and get a better night's sleep. Some people prefer taking their magnesium in divided doses, and that's OK. I prefer to take it all at once with my evening meal. There are also topical magnesium supplements and you can give those a try.

NIAGEN

Niagen is a form of vitamin B3 that helps to increase NAD+ levels in the human body, which is critical for cellular processes, metabolic pathways, and the maintenance and repair of DNA. I was originally turned on to Niagen as a way to decrease recovery time in between sets while working out—and it worked! I am now finding out that Niagen has a host of anti-aging benefits.

According to their website, these benefits include:

Healthy Aging: by supporting cellular function and metabolism.

Cellular Energy: by fueling your body's energy engines—the mitochondria.

Cellular Defense: by helping cells defend against metabolic stresses.

Cellular Repair: by promoting repair at the cellular level, counteracting the effects of stress.

An article from the *Life Extension Foundation* claimed that Niagen helped to protect your DNA from damage, but more research needs to be done to verify this. Although I only started taking Niagen for workout purposes, I now consider it a vital part of my anti-aging strategy. I feel the difference when I am on it and previous *Fat Loss After 40* clients have glowing things to say about it. If I was independently wealthy, I would take 500 mg of Niagen every day and an extra 500 mg on workout days. I am currently taking 300 mg every day, and on workout days I add 100 mg.

What it looks like:

In short, you could look at this through the lens of breakfast, lunch, and dinner. For breakfast take your vitamin D, if there is no sun available to you, and Niagen. For lunch (or breakfast) you can take your omega-3 / L-carnitine / ubiquinol stack. You need to have a meal containing healthy fats for the ubiquinol to be properly absorbed. (Because ubiquinol can increase cellular energy, do not take it with dinner as it might keep you up at night.) For dinner, take your magnesium with your meal.

That's it! Simple, yet powerful.

MY SECRET MORNING STACK

Note: If you do not consume caffeine then do not start; however, if you drink coffee and would like an alternative, then you may benefit from my secret morning stack.

In Chinese medicine, herbal formulas have a hierarchy. Certain herbs are the "king" herb and others are the "assistants" that help to enhance or counteract any undesired effects of the king herb. My morning stack is designed to be taken first thing in the morning with a bottle of water.

The main component is guarana, which is a South American herb that has naturally occurring caffeine. I take a standardized formula that provides 200 mg of naturally occurring caffeine. The main difference between taking coffee and a guarana tablet is that coffee hits you fast and comes down fast, at which point most people will consume another cup of coffee—until they look back and realize they have drunk six to eight cups of coffee in a day. A guarana tablet on the other hand comes on a little bit slower but lasts a longer time with an even keel; thus, instead of constantly taking "hits" of caffeine, taking the tablet allows for an energy plateau of about four to five hours.

The first assistant is L-theanine, and I will usually consume a 200–400 mg dose, depending on the day and intention. Most of the time it is a 200 mg dose and what it does is take the jitteriness away from the caffeine and allow you to concentrate better. If I want to meditate for a longer time, I will take a higher dose. Without L-theanine I can meditate for fifteen minutes, with L-theanine, I can meditate for forty-five minutes, and with a "double dose" of L-theanine, I can meditate for ninety minutes.

The next assistant component is DHA or MCT oil. While it is true that omega-3s are better consumed with foods, in this particular case, I am adding DHA to serve as "fuel" for the caffeine and allow it to burn more cleanly. The best metaphor I can use is that when I add the omega-3s or MCTs to the caffeine, my brain feels like a dry sponge that was allowed to "reabsorb water." The fat makes your brain and caffeine work better.

The fourth component, which is optional, is the addition of a specific modifier, which can be anything from ginkgo biloba to increase circulation in the brain, theacrine to increase energy, to any other nootropic like adrafinil, noopept, racetams (piracetam, aniracetam, oxiracetam), etc. to increase performance. This fourth component allows you to experiment with different compounds to get different effects and keep the morning stack varied and exciting. In my case, I add 300 mg of Niagen to the morning stack.

Thanks to this stack, I have not consumed coffee in over *twenty years*.

PART IV

PREP FOR SUCCESS

CHAPTER 8

SUCCESS TIPS

There are multiple ways to be successful with the *Fat Loss After 40* program. You can employ some or all of what I have included in this book. An accountability partner can be helpful at every level. And a coach can be invaluable, making sure you stick to the program and get the results you are looking for.

If your goal is to lose ten pounds:

- Report to an accountability partner daily with your morning weight
- Follow a Carnivore Diet

Being able to follow through just on this level should grant you success in thirty days or less.

If your goal is to lose ten to fifteen pounds:

- Report to an accountability partner daily with your morning weight
- Follow a thirty-day Carnivore Experiment
- Finish the month with a Liver Cleanse

If your goal is to lose thirty to forty-five pounds:

- Report to an accountability partner (or coach) daily with your morning weight
- Follow a thirty-day Carnivore Experiment
- Perform one Liver Cleanse a month until you reach your goal
- After the first month, you can stay on the Carnivore Diet or start adding other foods; the morning weight will show you how that food affects your weight
- Incorporate fasting and be able to finish a 24-, 48-, and finally a 72-hour fast over a three-month period
- Begin a workout program that is right for you and where you are in life right now
- Improve your sleep with the tips included; aim for seven to eight hours a night
- Ensure your nutrition is on point with the supplements mentioned
- Look at this as a three-to-four-month goal
- You will likely require a coach

You will also need a coach if you have any condition that requires a "workaround." This includes an injury or condition which prevents you from doing certain movements. A good coach will find an alternate way to get you there and, if done correctly, then "all roads lead to Rome."

When selecting a coach, the three most important qualities to look for are:

First and foremost, is your coach "technically and tactically proficient," as they say in the military? In other words, is your prospective coach a *living embodiment* of what you are hiring him or her for?

You would not hire a bodybuilding coach to help you win an interpretive dance contest, and you would not hire an interpretive dance coach to help you win an Ironman Triathlon.

Now that you get the principle, what does that mean?

Well, is your coach over forty, fit, and well-versed in the myriad of metabolic, endocrine, and soft tissue pain issues that come with being over forty? Is he or she able to modify exercises or principles to meet some of your unique needs or work around pain or injuries?

Second, and almost as important as the first one, how much does your coach *care*?

Are you just another number or are you a valued friend and client?

There is an old adage that goes, "People don't care how much you know until they know how much you care." I have found this to be true.

I know I "should" be more detached, but when I take on a client, I take it personally. When they "win," I feel great, and when they "slip," I immediately reach out and get them back on track, or I will agonize over it.

One way I do this is by limiting my client load so that I know everyone personally. I know their significant other's name and what they are going through, their kids if they have any, along with their professional and personal aspirations. You can't do this if you have too many clients at the same time.

Third, do they have a *track record of success*? In other words, have they coached anyone else to achieve what you want to achieve with them?

You would be surprised at how many people in the "fitness" industry do not have such a track record. Sure, they can write a convincing "article," but when pressed hard, there is no evidence that anybody ever trained with their methods.

DON'T BE FOOLED

Did you know that a lot of "fitness articles" are actually made up by fitness writers?

That's right!

A lot of "fitness magazines" come up with plausible workout scenarios, write a great story about it (which may or may not be true), and then hire a fitness model to do a photoshoot highlighting what you read in the article.

Maybe you already knew this, but I know I used to think that the pictures of the person in the article were a direct result of the training program I was reading about.

Nope!

Please be assured that the *Fat Loss After 40* program has been developed and constantly improved over a five-year period of working with real people all over the world (thanks to online coaching).

STICK WITH THE PROGRAM

When it comes to *Fat Loss After 40,* you want to have a support structure that helps you deal with setbacks, whether it is an injury or binging on a cruise and putting on eight extra pounds after you had successfully dropped five pounds.

Most people are "excited" about the program for about three days. After that, if you are alone, and no one is holding you accountable, it is too easy to give up at the first bump in the road.

Or you may fall prey to something that affects us all at one point or another, you read something else, and then you "switch strategies" without staying on one program long enough to squeeze all the benefits out of it.

If you jump from program to program, no progress will be made, and this is where you might throw in the towel. Further, well-meaning but ill-informed family and friends might encourage you to just "accept your age" and to "give up" these crazy notions of being fit at forty. If that is all you have to listen to, then the likelihood of you "dropping out" is very high.

However, if you have a good coach, the likelihood of you finishing the program and dropping the weight increases exponentially!

A good coach should be able to get you to the best version of yourself. Most people over forty are disconnected from their dreams. Perhaps they are stuck in a rut—physically, mentally, and financially—where every day is just a repetition of the previous one, and they have sacrificed all their dreams, hopes, and aspirations for the practicality of "paying the bills," "being a good provider," or "being a good husband and father (or wife and mother)."

While there is nothing "wrong" with being responsible and mature, there is nothing "right" about giving up on life and your dreams.

In the case of the *Fat Loss After 40* program, that means reconnecting with your childhood dreams and getting excited about your future.

A good coach should be able to bridge the gap from where you are now, which could be overweight and in pain, into a functionally fit human being capable of beginning any physical discipline you desire.

Remember, 80 percent of humans do *not* enjoy going to the gym!

Sure, you might do it out of necessity or as part of a New Year's resolution, but the truth of the matter is that you will not stick with something you don't like for very long.

You *can* stick to a gym or structured program for eight to twelve weeks if that liberates you to do something you truly enjoy—whether it be playing basketball, starting rock climbing, training for a marathon, or beginning mixed martial arts.

A good coach will believe in you before you believe it's possible for yourself.

Now, you have all the knowledge to achieve *Fat Loss After 40*—go out and change the world with your example!

CONCLUSION

Now you know the structure behind my *Fat Loss After 40* program. If you do nothing but follow the instructions for the first month and adopt a Carnivore Elimination Diet and do the Liver Cleanse at the end of that month, you will drop ten to fifteen pounds without exercise. If you wish to make this more achievable, I suggest getting an accountability partner—someone you have to check-in with *every day*. It could be someone doing the program with you or it could be someone you trust who will keep you honest.

Always remember that simplicity is the key to success in the *Fat Loss After 40* program. Sure, you can read the whole book from cover to cover in one sitting and sound smart at parties, or you can try to implement everything at once, or you can choose only those things you like and try them out at your leisure...*but*, if you truly want to achieve results with the *Fat Loss After 40* program then I would suggest sticking to the structured plan and taking it one month at a time:

FIRST MONTH

1. Mindset and the Carnivore Elimination Diet

2. Homozon and Sleep

3. Liver Cleanse

SECOND MONTH

1. Slo-mo Workout

2. Fasting 24-48-72

THIRD MONTH

1. Uphill Sprints to Boost HGH

2. Anti-Aging Stacks and Supplements

Your "graduation exercise" is connecting with the things that really *excite* you. What do I mean by that? Well, ask most people over forty who are struggling with weight issues what they want, and they respond with, "Oh, if I could just lose ten or twenty pounds, I would be happy."

However...,

Once they drop thirty to forty-five pounds, get out of pain, and restore functioning levels of strength, conditioning, flexibility, mobility, endurance, and agility, then the answers to that same question are very different. Then they see themselves as capable! The conversation is no longer about "settling" for ten or twenty pounds! It is about reconnecting to childhood dreams and desires.

Suddenly, the answers sound more like this:

"You know, I always wanted to participate in elite level rowing."

"Now that you mention it, I have always wanted to run a marathon, but just never felt I could."

"I would really like to do an Ironman once in my life."

"Ever since I was little I wanted to learn martial arts."

"I always wanted to hike the Grand Canyon or hike the Appalachian Trail."

"I want to compete in fencing."

"I want to learn parkour!"

Do you see the difference between settling for a couple of pounds versus connecting to your childhood dreams and desires? Once you regain your ability to be fit after forty with the *Fat Loss After 40* program, use it to live your *best life* and do the things you have always wanted to do.

I look forward to hearing about your success with the program!

SO, YOU'VE LOST 30-45 POUNDS... NOW WHAT?

Let's say you have followed the program for three months and lost 30-45 pounds. Do you go back to the way you were before?

Well, if you go back to your old ways, you are going to put the weight back on.

If you want to keep the weight off, then you are going to have to adopt a healthy lifestyle.

No, it does not mean you have to be "perfect" or become

Carnivore 24/7, but it does mean that you need some sort of structure that serves you and keeps you on track.

I have known people that like to "let themselves go" and take three months to drop the extra weight. They like to eat and drink with gusto and then "suck it up" for three months every year. While you could do that, that is not my preferred recommendation for the Fat Loss After 40 program.

Here is what I do on a regular basis to remain "combat ready"—I eat two meals a day.

My first meal is protein and fat. It could be steak, eggs, burger patties, sausage, or any combination thereof.

My second meal is a regular meal containing carbs, protein, and fat. This one could be as simple as steak, veggies, and rice. If I am hungry, I will have seconds. I don't count calories, and I have plenty of "cheat days."

Here is what I do at least once a year—I do a 30-day Carnivore reset and a liver cleanse, usually in January since most of us tend to overeat during Thanksgiving and Christmas holidays, to include a lot of sugary snacks.

I started doing this because I noticed that one of the biggest factors affecting aging and weight gain is that every year people tend to put on weight after the holidays and that weight never seems to come off. After ten to twenty years, they look in the mirror and don't recognize themselves.

By starting the year with a 30-day Carnivore reset and a liver cleanse, you nip this tendency right in the bud and start the year without the holiday weight gain.

I too put on weight during the holidays! The only difference is that while people were recovering from their hangovers after New Year's Day, I would do a liver cleanse and return to work five pounds lighter.

One way to look at life post *Fat Loss After 40* is to follow the visual recommendations by Frank Suarez in his book *The Power of Your Metabolism.* He developed a simple and elegant system for weight management. He calls it the 2x1 or the 3x1 system. In a nutshell, in the 2x1 system, you divide your plate into three equal portions. Two portions are to be your protein/fat source (chicken, fish, meat) and veggies, one portion of the plate is the carbs. In this system, no food is off limits, and this seems to resonate with a lot of people.

Of course, if you want to lose weight faster, you can implement a 3x1 system in which you divide the plate into four equal portions and eat three portions of meats and veggies and only one portion (or 25 percent of the plate) in carbs.

This system works by controlling insulin. If you want to

really understand how controlling insulin through dietary changes can help you then I highly recommend you get his book.

If you are having trouble sleeping, then you might want to look at cortisol. For this I recommend the book *The Adrenal Reset Diet* by Alan Christianson, NMD. His main point is that you want to cycle carbs to manage cortisol. You want to minimize carbs in the morning so cortisol can spike, and you want to consume carbs in the evening so cortisol can go down and melatonin can come up.

Now you have an off-ramp from the Fat Loss After 40 program that you can live with, so that you can keep the weight off.

Should you ever put on a few pounds, then it's nothing that a Carnivore reset and a liver cleanse can't fix and put you back on track.

The other important point is to find a physical activity that you like and enjoy doing. While the Slo-mo workout and Uphill Sprints are great, most people do not enjoy working out and will not stick to it long term.

However, most people can stick to a physical activity they do like. Maybe you start surfing, kayaking, or hiking up mountains, or perhaps you double-down and join a master's league of a sport you have played in your youth. Having an active lifestyle is not about hitting the weights in the gym, even though there is nothing wrong with that. It's about, well, having an active lifestyle!

Only you know what excites you and keeps you pumped up.

You now have a new lease on life! Don't waste it, use it to the best of your ability!

FURTHER RESEARCH

The Joe Rogan Experience podcast with Jordan Peterson on Carnivore Diet

The Joe Rogan Experience podcast with Mikhaela Peterson on Carnivore Diet

The Carnivore Diet by Dr. Shawn Baker

Lies My Doctor Told Me by Dr. Ken Berry

The Adrenal Reset Diet by Alan Christianson, NMD

The Power of Your Metabolism by Frank Suarez

The Self-Reliance Manifesto by Eric Guttmann

Wheat Belly by Dr. William Davis

Fast and Grow Young by Herbert Shelton

The Healing Sun by Richard Hobday

Defending Beef by Nicolette Hahn Niman

Can't Hurt Me by David Goggins

Flood Your Body with Oxygen by Ed McCabe

ACKNOWLEDGMENTS

First and foremost, I have to thank my wife Vianca for always believing in me! She was the first to tell me, "Stop buying other people's books and start writing your own." She is my most trusted confidante and absolute best friend in life.

My kids, Max, Eric, Oscar, and Vianca Patricia for being the "light" of my life and being with me in this journey every step of the way. When I needed strength to carry me through all the challenges in the last twenty years, I knew I had to because of you guys.

While the list of coaches who have influenced me over the past forty years is vast, there are three who really stand out when it comes to *Fat Loss After 40*.

Stephen Santangelo is as close to a "national treasure" as any American can hope to be. During our many conversations, I am able to take a single concept and extract incredible value from it. For example, during our talks, he mentioned that one of the keys to fat loss was to "avoid spiking insulin in the morning." That one comment prompted me to experiment with things that led to creating *Fat Loss After 40*.

Eric Fiorillo was the strongman behind the *Motivation and Muscle* podcast. The actual term *Fat Loss After 40* was born out of one of his podcasts where he interviewed me on this subject. That one podcast led to an online course, a private coaching program, and now a book! Eric, I know you are watching from above, and I am truly grateful to have had the honor and privilege of knowing you while you walked the earth. I am sure you are lifting heavy stones in heaven to your heart's content.

Matt Furey is a coach and friend who is well-known in the health and fitness industry. I have known Matt since 2004, and I have become a better coach by observing him. I learned the value of daily accountability from him. He was also the person who got me to try my first thirty-day Carnivore experiment by asking me if "I wanted to see if I was addicted to food." Matt, your talk on "emotional energy" upon leaving the military was a great kindness at a time when it was sorely needed. Thank you.

I learned the two questions to screen applicants from Ed Strachar.

Dick Sutphen and Robert Fritz for combining elements I learned from them into the mindset exercise for *Fat Loss After 40*.

I have a huge debt of gratitude to Sophie May, Chas Hoppe, Laura Cail, and all the wonderful people at Scribe Media who were able to take this project all the way to the finish line. The book you now hold in your hands is a testament to their work ethic and professionalism.

Finally, and most importantly, to every person who has ever served...*Thank You!*

Made in the USA
Columbia, SC
13 July 2023

20370858R00071